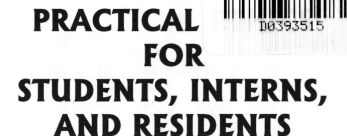

PRACTICAL
FOR
STUDENTS, INTERNS,
AND RESIDENTS

A Short Reference Manual

Second Edition

Charles Junkerman, M.D.
Professor Emeritus
Department of Medicine
Center for the Study of Bioethics
Medical College of Wisconsin

David Schiedermayer, M.D.
Associate Professor
Division of General Internal Medicine
Department of Medicine
Medical College of Wisconsin

For Anne and Kim,
practical ethicists in our residences

University Publishing Group, Inc.
Hagerstown, Maryland 21740
1-800-654-8188

ISBN 1-55572-054-4

CONTENTS

INTRODUCTION

The concepts described here are as important to patient care as any diagnostic or management techniques. Evaluative strategies and therapeutic interventions will change frequently, but if the physician-in-training can master the art of communication with patients and can learn to identify and resolve ethical problems, he or she will have acquired enduring, career-enhancing skills.

This text contains a brief overview of the information needed to provide comprehensive, ethical, patient-centered care. In this revised edition, new sections on futility, assisted suicide, and managed care have been added. Each section contains concise information on the topic listed. Many of the sections include additional material and a list of a few important references for those who wish to pursue further a given subject.

ACKNOWLEDGMENTS

Many residents in medicine and fellow faculty members at the Medical College of Wisconsin reviewed the text and provided valuable suggestions. The authors are especially appreciative of the encouragement offered by our editor, Ms. Leslie LeBlanc, and of her support for a short, physician-friendly ethics manual. The early assistance of Dr. Mahendr S. Kochar, Professor of Medicine and Associate Dean for Graduate Medical Education, was invaluable. Review by Dr. Mark Adams, Dr. Carl Chan, Dr. Elsa Cohen, Dr. Arthur Derse, Dr. William Greaves, Dr. Robert Nelson, Dr. David Weissman, Ms. Sandy Pasch, and Attorney Robyn Shapiro has enhanced the accuracy of particular sections and is greatly appreciated. Dr. Rebekah Wang-Cheng supplied much of the text for the section on difficult patients. Thorough review and cogent comments by our colleagues at other institutions—Dr. Dale Berg, Dr. John La Puma, and Dr. Kenneth Simpson—have resulted in a more readable text. The ongoing support and encouragement of Dr. Rick Lofgren, Chief, Division of General Internal Medicine, is gratefully acknowledged.

I. DO NOT RESUSCITATE (DNR)

DISCUSSION WITH THE PATIENT

The issue of cardiopulmonary resuscitation (CPR) should be addressed early in the treatment course of a patient with serious illness in whom cardiac or pulmonary arrest is likely. The subject should be approached sensitively as part of the overall therapeutic plan. The comfort and therapeutic measures that will remain in effect should be emphasized and discussed first.

AUTHORITY FOR DNR

Legal authority for the decision (in order of importance):

1. Request of a decisional patient (a patient who has decision-making capacity; see section IV)
2. Dictates of an advance directive
3. Judgment of guardian or healthcare agent appointed in an advance directive.

In some states, surrogate laws establish a hierarchy of authority; in others, there is moral authority but no legal authority for the following (if 1 to 3 above are not available):

4. Approval by first-order relatives (spouse, adult children, or parents—in that order)
5. Opinions of other relatives or friends who are able to provide a "substituted judgment" (section IV, page 18) or who agree upon the best interest of the patient
6. If no relatives or friends are available for consultation, base the decision on medical indications, taking into account whether CPR would further the reasonable personal medical goals of this particular patient.

WHAT THE DNR ORDER SHOULD INCLUDE

1. The order should be written by the attending physician or by a house officer at the request of the attending physician.

2. Documentation in the progress note of:
   - The medical indication for DNR or contraindication to CPR
   - Advice of consultants (if any)
   - Authority for the decision (see above discussion).
3. Specific orders about what treatments are to continue. Specific orders should be in writing to avoid misunderstandings. Ordinarily, DNR simply means "no CPR." DNR may have no other significance and may be compatible with all other modalities of treatment including care in the intensive care unit. On the other hand, a DNR order may be the first step in the withdrawal of other treatment, in which case further clarification is necessary.

DNR ORDERS ON THE BASIS OF FUTILITY

In many institutions, a DNR order may be written on the basis of medical futility (see section IX, page 28). Another staff physician should concur in writing, and the justification for this judgment must be clearly indicated in the progress notes. Many policies stipulate that the patient or surrogate need not agree but must be notified. If the patient or surrogate disagrees with the decision, consultation with the institutional ethics committee is appropriate and hospital administration should be notified.

DISCUSSION WITH THE NURSING STAFF

The rationale and specific orders need to be discussed fully with the nursing staff and the patient's other caregivers so that there are no uncertainties about care plans. Patients are either DNR as clearly specified in the orders or they are full code. "Slow codes," "code grays," "show codes," or "Hollywood codes" are deceptive and place an unfair responsibility on the nursing service.

ATTENTION TO TLC

Many patients and their families fear abandonment when a DNR order is written, so it is important for physicians and nurses to be more attentive and aware of comfort measures. The patient and family must know from the outset that "no code" does not mean "no care."

ETHICS CONSULTATION

In the event that the authority for DNR is in question or a DNR order written on the basis of futility has created objections on the part of patient, family, or agent, an ethics consultation should be sought for clarification or mediation.

FURTHER READING

CPR was developed in the 1960s for treatment of sudden cardiac arrest in previously well individuals. Despite warnings that this technique could be inappropriate in other clinical situations, CPR became a default procedure. It was presumed that a patient wanted CPR unless there was a specific request to avoid it. This is a unique presumption in medicine.

Effectiveness of CPR

Public expectations of the success of CPR are quite unrealistic and do not match the statistics. About 15 percent of hospitalized patients in whom resuscitation is attempted survive to discharge. Furthermore, numerous studies have shown virtually no survival to hospital discharge for patients with overwhelming pneumonia, renal failure, acute stroke, or multiple organ failure who have an in-hospital arrest. Patients over 70 years of age who have sepsis or metastatic carcinoma or whose resuscitation effort lasts more than 15 minutes are unlikely to survive. Recent research suggests, however, that CPR success varies from one institution to another and that the pre-arrest condition of the patient may be the most important predictor of success.

The best CPR results occur in persons who have a witnessed arrest on the basis of a ventricular dysrhythmia (not asystole) and who are successfully resuscitated within five minutes. CPR is successful in 25 percent of cardiac arrests that result from drug reaction or overdose. Extended CPR (more than 15 minutes) is reasonable in cases of subarachnoid hemorrhage, hypothermia, electric shock, and drug overdose.

Risks (Burdens) of CPR

Of the patients who are successfully resuscitated, 25 to 50 percent have fractured ribs, fractured sternum, aspiration pneumonia, mediastinal hemorrhage, or pulmonary edema. Up to 10 percent of those whose CPR is successful may end up in a persistent vegetative state.

Discussion with the Patient

When to talk about CPR with a patient is a matter of clinical judgment. For example, this discussion is probably unnecessary in the case of a healthy woman entering the hospital in labor or a healthy young man coming in for a hernia repair. There is no need to unduly alarm such patients. Furthermore, for such patients the desire for CPR and the prospect of a successful outcome can reasonably be presumed in the unlikely event of a catastrophe requiring resuscitation.

The discussion is mandatory, however, when patients are admitted for serious illnesses in which an arrest would not be unlikely or when patients have chronic illnesses and their condition may deteriorate. The wishes of these patients cannot be presumed and, therefore, should be elicited.

Questions about the patient's desire for CPR need to be asked in the specific context of that patient's problems. One should avoid questions such as "Do you want us to do everything?" when "everything" is practically impossible for the patient or physician to define. Likewise, the question "Do you want us to start your heart if it stops?" implies falsely that such a result may be certain.

The issue should be approached sensitively and as a part of the overall therapeutic program. The patient may need more information in order to make a decision. The physician should provide this information, along with some indication of whether CPR is recommended for this particular patient in this particular context. If the patient desires or the situation dictates, a more extensive discussion about the likely success and the burdens and risks of CPR should ensue.

If CPR would likely be futile (see section IX), a request for a DNR order should probably follow a discussion emphasizing the positive measures that will be taken for the patient, the reassurance that the patient will not be abandoned, and the promise that all possible comfort measures will be provided. The physician can say that CPR is not a reasonable part of the patient's specific treatment "package." "We are not giving up on you; we are giving up on some treatment strategies that won't work and are not in your best interest."

Some ethicists advocate, with good reason, that DNR should be DNAR (do not attempt resuscitation) because DNR implies that a reasonable degree of success is possible. In patients for whom a DNR or no-CPR order is appropriate, the likelihood of success is usually minimal. To imply otherwise is to mislead the patient and thereby impair his or her autonomous judgment.

If some unforeseen event takes place in the hospital that makes cardiac or pulmonary arrest likely, the subject of code status should be brought up while the patient still has decision-making capacity (if possible). It is not ethical to wait purposefully until an acutely ill patient is no longer decisional in order to discuss code status with a surrogate.

Conflict between the Patient's Desire for "Full Code" and Futility

The American Medical Association (AMA) Council on Judicial and Ethical Affairs has commented that resuscitative efforts "would be considered futile if they could not be expected to achieve the goals expressed by the informed patient. This definition of futility not only respects the autonomy and value judgments of individual patients but also allows for the professional judgment and guidance of physicians who render care to patients" (*JAMA*. 1991;265:1868-1871).

Occasionally patients in whom CPR is almost certain to fail insist on the attempt. If the request is clearly irrational (for example, a patient wishes CPR not in an attempt to survive until the arrival of a loved one but simply as part of wanting "everything" done), the physician is under no obligation to provide futile treatment. This right is recognized in law and ethics. Strategies for avoiding this conflict between the patient's desire for futile treatment and the physician's reluctance to use a treatment that is not medically indicated include the following:

1. Avoid using the term *futility*, which is hard to define and even more difficult for patients to understand.
2. Determine the patient's goals in the present circumstances.
3. Determine in discussion with the patient or surrogate whether an attempt at resuscitation in light of its benefits and burdens will further these goals.

Relationship of DNR to Advance Directives (ADs)

DNR orders should not be confused with advance directives. ADs require interpretation and need to be incorporated into a treatment plan that includes specific orders consistent with the patient's wishes. This plan may or may not include a DNR order, but DNR is not usually a part of the AD. The existence of a living will does not necessarily indicate that a patient is intent on forgoing CPR.

DNR and the Operating Room (OR)

Anesthesiologists have expressed their discomfort with DNR orders in the OR because an arrest might occur during a procedure in the OR that is not related to the underlying disease, and this arrest may be easily managed with drugs. In this situation, anesthesiologists are reluctant to stand by and watch the patient die. Therefore, DNR policies should be modified so that ordinarily the DNR order is suspended when the patient goes to the OR (or a procedure such as cardiac catheterization) and is reinstituted automatically on discharge from the recovery room. The patient should be notified of the policy for placing the DNR order on hold and should have the option of overriding the policy, keeping the DNR order in effect through the procedure.

REFERENCES

American Medical Association, Council on Ethical and Judicial Affairs. Guidelines for appropriate use of do-not-resuscitate orders. *JAMA*. 1991;265:1868-1871.

Hakim RB, et al. Factors associated with do-not-resuscitate orders: patients' preferences, prognoses, and physicians' judgments. *Ann Intern Med*. 1996;125:284-293.

Jayes RL, et al. Do-not-resuscitate orders in intensive care units. *JAMA*. 1993;270:2213-2217.

Kane RS, Burns EA. Cardiopulmonary resuscitation policies in long term care facilities. *J Am Geriatric Soc*. 1997;45:154-157.

Lo B. Unanswered questions about DNR orders. *JAMA*. 1991;265:1874-1875.

Loewy EH. Changing one's mind: when is Odysseus to be believed? *J Gen Intern Med*. 1988;3:54-58.

Tomlinson T, Brody H. Futility and the ethics of resuscitation. *JAMA*. 1990;264:1276-1280.

Walker RM. DNR in the OR: resuscitation as an operative risk. *JAMA*. 1991;266:2407-2412.

Wenger NS, et al. Patients with DNR orders in the operating room: surgery, resuscitation, and outcomes. *J Clin Ethics*. 1997;8:250-257.

II. WITHDRAWAL OF TREATMENT

AUTHORITY FOR WITHDRAWAL OF TREATMENT
Authority for the decision (in order of importance):
1. Request of a decisional patient (section IV, page 16)
2. Dictates of an advance directive
3. Judgment of guardian or healthcare agent appointed in an advance directive
4. Approval of relatives (spouse, adult children, parents, and adult siblings—in that order; order established by surrogate laws in some states and by convention in others)
5. Approval of close friends who know the patient's treatment preferences or are able to make decisions that promote the patient's best interest.

DIFFERENCE BETWEEN WITHDRAWING AND WITHHOLDING
1. Psychological Difference
Psychologically, it is easier not to start a treatment than it is to stop it. But a moment's reflection demonstrates that this is illogical—the decision to omit treatment is just as much a willful judgment as the decision to withdraw it.
2. "Up-Front Barrier"
When we decide not to start a specific treatment, we may be erecting an "up-front barrier"—that is, we may be denying in advance a treatment that might possibly be effective. Thus, a decision not to initiate treatment (to withhold treatment) must actually have stronger substantiating reasons than a decision to discontinue (withdraw) treatment that has clearly failed.
3. Time-Limited Trial
When there is some uncertainty as to the effectiveness of a treatment in furthering the patient's goals, the bias clearly must be in favor of a time-limited trial of treatment. If it later

turns out to be ineffective and not beneficial for a particular patient in a given circumstance, the treatment can be stopped. By using this model, we have given the patient a reasonable chance of attaining the goals of a specific therapy.

WITHDRAWAL OF VENTILATORS
1.   Patients with Brain Death

When the criteria for brain death have been satisfied (section VII, page 23), the person is legally dead and there is no obligation to continue ventilation. The ventilator may be removed as soon as the pronouncement of death has been entered into the chart. Organ donation and sensitivity to the family's needs may legitimately delay this procedure for several hours.

2.   Sentient Patients
Method of Withdrawal

When the decision has been made to remove a ventilator from a patient who is (or could be presumed to be) conscious and aware of the consequences, there is no good reason for weaning (the gradual decrease of ventilatory support), as the process often results in dyspnea and a sense of suffocation. After adequate sedation, the ventilator should be discontinued abruptly. Whether the endotracheal tube should be removed or remain in place for suctioning involves a judgment call.

Sedation

Before the ventilator is removed, the patient should be sedated heavily with a benzodiazepine or a barbiturate and morphine in doses adequate to produce unconsciousness but not sufficient to produce death. The sedation should be continued until death has occurred. It requires the clinical judgment of the physician at the bedside to know how much and how long to sedate the patient in order to avoid further suffering.

Paralyzing Agents

Under no circumstances should respiratory paralyzing agents be initiated during ventilator withdrawal because such agents hinder evaluation of the patient's suffering and discomfort. However, if a patient is already on these agents, it is not necessary to wait until the drug is entirely cleared from the system to begin the process of sedation and ventilator withdrawal.

WITHDRAWAL OF FLUID AND NUTRITION

1. Patients in a Persistent Vegetative State (PVS)

In many states, living will statutes allow persons to state that they do not want fluid and nutrition if they are in a PVS (see section VIII, page 25). Such support can be withdrawn from these patients without causing suffering because, by definition, the symptoms of thirst and hunger are cortically mediated and cannot be present.

2. Sentient Patients

Decision to Withdraw

In many states, power of attorney for healthcare laws specifically allow a person to give the agent the authority to withhold or to withdraw a feeding tube, regardless of whether the patient is in a PVS. The decisional patient, of course, retains the right to refuse artificially provided fluid and nutrition.

Effect of Withdrawal

When both food and fluid are withdrawn, death usually occurs from electrolyte imbalance and dehydration in 10 to 14 days. If fluid is maintained and food withdrawn, death occurs from starvation and may take many weeks. For this reason, both food and fluid should be withdrawn or withheld. Patients are rarely uncomfortable in the clinical situations in which food and fluid are likely to be withdrawn. Ice chips and good oral care can assuage symptoms of dry mouth and provide comfort care.

Intravenous (IV) Access

Occasionally IV access is needed for palliative drug administration. A "keep-open" rate will not provide sufficient fluid to prolong the dying process significantly.

FURTHER READING

Rights of the Decisional Patient

The courts have made important statements on the rights of patients to decide about medical treatment. Justice B.N. Cardozo wrote in 1914, "Every human being of adult years and sound mind has a right to determine what shall be done with his own body" (Katz. 1972;526). The *Bartling* decision in California found that "Competent adult patients with serious illnesses which are probably incurable but have not been diagnosed as terminal have the right over the objections of their physicians and the hospital to have life support equipment disconnected despite the fact that withdrawal of such devices will surely hasten death."

Differences between Medical Treatment and Supportive Care

Important differences exist between medical treatment and supportive care. *Medical treatment* is provided by physicians and other health professionals; it is aimed at accomplishing the goals of medical practice. *Supportive care* can be provided by heath professionals but is often provided by other caregivers such as family members; it is aimed at providing comfort to the dying patient. Providing human comfort is imperative, but no "technological imperative" exists. Thus, healthcare professionals are not obligated to provide specialized, life-sustaining treatment to every patient simply because such technology is available.

Difference between Withdrawing and Withholding

The President's Commission for the Study of Ethical Problems in Medicine and Biomedical and Behavioral Research noted in 1982 that the distinction between withholding (failing to initiate) therapy and withdrawing (discontinuing) therapy was not of moral importance. The commission believed that a justification adequate for not commencing a treatment was sufficient for ceasing a treatment that proved ineffective and noted that erecting a higher requirement for cessation might discourage trials of treatments that might sometimes be successful.

Right to Withdrawal of Fluid and Nutrition

Some controversy has existed about whether administration of food and fluid through a feeding tube is a medical treatment or "ordinary care." This has effectively been settled by two court decisions.

In *In re L.W.* (1992), the Wisconsin Supreme Court cited the New Jersey *Conroy* decision (1985), which acknowledged the emotional significance of food but noted that feeding by implanted tubes is a medical procedure with inherent risks and possible side effects, instituted by skilled healthcare providers to compensate for impaired physical functioning. The court noted that this procedure, analytically, is equivalent to artificial breathing using a respirator.

In an opinion in the U.S. Supreme Court *Cruzan* case (1990), Justice Sandra Day O'Connor said, "Artificial feeding cannot readily be distinguished from other forms of medical treatment. The techniques used to pass food and water into the patient's alimentary tract all involve some degree of intrusion and restraint. Requiring a competent adult to endure such procedures against her will burdens the patient's liberty, dignity and freedom to determine the course of her own treatment."

Effect of Withdrawal of Fluid and Nutrition

Hypernatremia and hypercalcemia occur in many patients after withdrawal of fluid and nutrition. These changes, along with hyperosmolarity, azotemia, and increased endogenous opioids, often produce a sedative effect on the brain during the dying process. Hospice workers have provided other observations:

1. Persons near death often voluntarily stop eating and drinking and do not tolerate substantial volumes of enteral feedings.
2. Dying persons who are given "normal" replacement fluids commonly show signs of fluid overload, including distressing pulmonary edema.
3. Despite substantial physiological deficits, hospice patients almost never report feeling hunger or thirst. Dry mouth and lips are easily remedied by lubricants and ice chips.
4. Dehydration results in less vomiting and diarrhea, less need to suction secretions, and less dyspnea and peripheral edema.

REFERENCES

ACCP/SCCM Consensus Panel. Ethical and moral guidelines for the initiation, continuation, and withdrawal of intensive care. *Chest*. 1990;97:949-958.

American Medical Association, Council on Ethical and Judicial Affairs. Decisions near the end of life. *JAMA*. 1992;267:2229-2233.

American Thoracic Society. Withholding and withdrawing life-sustaining therapy. *Ann Intern Med*. 1991;115:478 484.

Bartling v. Superior Court. 209 CalRptr 220;163 Cal App 3d(1986).

Brody H, Campbell ML, Faber-Langendoen K, Ogle KS. Withdrawing intensive life-sustaining treatments: recommendations for a compassionate clinical management. *N Engl J Med*. 1997;336:652-657.

Cruzan v. Missouri Dept of Health. 497 US; 111LEd 2d 224, 110 SCt 2841 (1990).

Hodges MO, Tolle SW. Tube feeding decisions in the elderly. *Clin in Geriatric Med*. 1994;10:475-488.

Katz J. *Experimentation with Human Beings*. New York: Russell Sage Foundation; 1972.

McCann RM, Hall WJ, Groth-Juncker A. Comfort care for terminally ill patients; the appropriate use of nutrition and hydration. *JAMA*. 1994;272:1263-1266.

Meisel A. Legal myths about terminating life support. *Arch Intern Med*. 1991;151:1497- 1502.

President's Commission for the Study of Ethical Problems in Medicine and Biomedical and Behavioral Research. *Deciding to Forego Life-Sustaining Treatment: Ethical, Medical and Legal Issues in Treatment Decisions*. Washington, DC: US Government Printing Office; 1983.

Printz LA. Terminal dehydration, a compassionate treatment. *Arch Intern Med*. 1992;152:697-700.

Ruark JE, Raffin TA. Initiating and withdrawing life support principles and practice in adult medicine. *N Engl J Med*. 1988;318:25-30.

III. INFORMED CONSENT

PURPOSE
The purpose of informed consent is to provide the patient with all of the information necessary to allow a reasonable person to make a prudent treatment choice on his or her own behalf.

ADEQUACY OF INFORMATION
According to the President's Commission for the Study of Ethical Problems in Medicine and Biomedical and Behavioral Research, adequate informed consent requires effort on the part of the physician to ensure comprehension; it involves far more than just a signature on the bottom of a list of possible complications. Such compilations can be so overwhelming that patients are unable to appreciate the truly significant information and to make sound decisions.

ELEMENTS OF INFORMED CONSENT
1. Information
The patient must have a clear understanding of:
   a. The disease process (diagnosis in understandable terms)
   b. Prognosis
   c. Benefits and burdens of recommended treatment
   d. Benefits and burdens of reasonable alternative treatments
   e. The likely effect of no treatment (this is always an option).

2. Consent
"Consent" is the patient's voluntary, autonomous authorization to proceed with the proposed intervention.

OBTAINING INFORMED CONSENT

Truly informed consent always involves the following elements:
1. Adequate disclosure of information
2. Decisional capacity of the patient
3. Patient's comprehension of the information
4. Voluntariness (freedom from coercion)
5. Consent of the patient.

DISCLOSURE STANDARDS USED BY THE COURTS

1. Professional Community Standard

What a capable and reasonable medical practitioner in the same field would reveal to a patient under the same or similar circumstances (some states use this standard).

2. Reasonable-Patient Standard

Because of doubt that a professional community standard can be identified, another standard has been developed, which asks for the information a reasonable patient would consider material to the decision of whether to consent to the procedure offered (some states use this standard).

EXCEPTIONS TO THE INFORMED CONSENT REQUIREMENT

1. Emergency Privilege

a. Patient must be unconscious, or without the capacity to make a decision, while no one legally authorized to act as agent for the patient is available.

b. Time must be of the essence, in the sense that there is a risk of serious bodily injury or death.

c. Under the circumstances, a reasonable person would consent.

2. **Therapeutic Privilege Disclosure Would Have an Adverse Effect on the Patient's Health**
   a. Must take into account the circumstances of the patient.
   b. Physician must believe that a full disclosure of the information will have a significantly adverse impact on the patient. (This standard has been much abused in the past; it should be used infrequently and with great discretion.)

3. **Patient Does Not Have Decisional Capacity**

   Patient must be decisional for consent to be informed or free.

4. **Waiver of Rights**

   Patient does not desire to have information. Physician should not force the issue but should document it well and ask for permission to inform a surrogate.

REFERENCES

Brody H. Transparency: informed consent in primary care. *Hastings Cent Rep*. 1989; 19(5): 5-9.

Meisel A, Kuczewski M. Legal and ethical myths about informed consent. *Arch Intern Med*. 1996;156:2521-2526.

President's Commission for the Study of Ethical Problems in Medicine and Biomedical and Behavioral Research. *Making Health Care Decisions: The Ethical and Legal Implications of Informed Consent in the Patient-Physician Relationship*. Washington, DC: US Government Printing Office; 1982.

IV. COMPETENCE AND DECISION-MAKING CAPACITY

DEFINITIONS

1. Competence

Competence and *incompetence* are legal terms. Technically, a patient remains competent until a court says otherwise.

2. Decision-Making Capacity

The determination of decision-making capacity can be made by medical personnel and does not require a court hearing.

CLINICAL ASSESSMENT OF DECISION-MAKING CAPACITY

In assessing a patient's ability to make autonomous judgments, one must evaluate the three distinct aspects of decision-making capacity:

1. Ability to Understand

- The ability to comprehend the given information about diagnosis and treatment and to identify the issue at hand (To test this, ask the patient to paraphrase the discussion.)
- The ability to appreciate the impact of the disease and its consequences (To test this, ask the patient to state the major options and the most likely outcome for each option.)

2. Ability to Evaluate

- The ability to deliberate in accordance with one's own values
- The ability to manipulate information rationally and to compare risks and benefits of the options
- The ability to make choices that are not irrational and to give the reasons for them
- The ability to maintain a consistent choice over time.

3. **Ability to Communicate**
   - The ability to communicate choices. (To test this, ask the patient to state his or her choice of treatment options.)

If the patient demonstrates satisfactory responses in all three areas, he or she is said to have "decision-making capacity," to be "decisional," or to be "capacitated."

DEGREE OF CONFIDENCE IN PATIENT'S DECISION-MAKING CAPACITY

1. If there is a favorable expectation from the patient's choice (little risk, large benefit), then a relatively low level of decision-making capacity is required.
2. If there is a balance of risk and benefit from the patient's choice, then a moderate level of decision-making capacity is required.
3. If expectations from the patient's choice are not favorable (great risk with little chance of benefit), then a high level of decision-making capacity is necessary.

THE MATURE MINOR

By legal definition, minors (under the age of 18 in most states) are not competent to make major healthcare decisions. Many states give minors limited autonomy; they are specifically allowed to obtain contraception, abortion, and treatment for venereal disease or substance abuse without parental permission. In many states, minors who are married or living independently and supporting themselves are considered to be "emancipated minors" and competent to make their own healthcare decisions. Moreover, developing case law on the "mature minor" now recognizes that as the adolescent's age increases toward maturity, he or she should have a progressively greater part in the decision-making process.

DECISION MAKING FOR INCAPACITATED PATIENTS

When a surrogate acts for an incapacitated patient, the basis for decision is one of the following:

1.   Substituted Judgment

This is the guideline the surrogate uses if the patient has expressed a preference before becoming incompetent, or if the surrogate knows the patient well enough to determine what the patient would choose if he or she were still decisional.

2.   Best Interest

This is the standard the surrogate must use when he or she has no clear idea of what the patient might choose. It is what a reasonable person might choose in the same context and is based on what is ultimately best for this particular patient in these particular circumstances.

When a patient has a legal guardian, this individual has the right to refuse life-sustaining treatment based on the patient's best interest in the light of the diagnosis, prognosis, and medical goals of treatment.

DIFFICULTIES IN MAKING JUDGMENTS FOR THE INCAPACITATED PATIENT

There are several complications in making ethical decisions that are in the best interest of an incapacitated patient.

1. We do not know the wishes of the patient in regard to the withdrawal of life-sustaining treatment in the context of the immediate clinical situation.

2. Since we do not have the autonomous wishes of the incompetent patient to act upon, we must rely on surrogates and professionals to make these decisions.

3. It is preferable to make quality-of-life judgments based on the patient's own assessment. Because incompetent patients cannot provide this information, quality-of-life determinations become subjective on the part of others—a risky evaluation at best.

REFERENCES

Cohen LM, McCue JD, Green GM. Do clinical and formal assessments of the capacity of patients in the intensive care unit to make decisions agree? *Arch Intern Med.* 1993;153;2481-2485.

Drane JF. Competency to give informed consent: a model for making clinical assessments. *JAMA*. 1984; 252:925-927.

Emmanuel EJ. What criteria should guide decision makers for incompetent patients? *Lancet*. 1988;1:170-171.

Miles SH, Koepp R, Weber EP. Advance end-of-life treatment planning. *Arch Intern Med*. 1996;156:1062-1068.

Schneiderman LJ, Arras, JD. Counseling patients to counsel physicians on future care in the event of patient incompetence. *Ann Intern Med*. 1985;102:693-698.

V. CONFIDENTIALITY

The patient's confidence that information given to the physician will remain private is an important element in the doctor-patient encounter. Without such assurance, the patient might be unwilling to divulge information critical to his or her care.

BASIS FOR THE PRINCIPLE
1. Inherent respect for an individual's privacy and autonomy
2. Special trust relationship in the doctor-patient encounter
3. Element of promise in the Hippocratic Oath
4. The good of society
5. Prevention of harm to the patient.

EXCEPTIONS
There may be legal exceptions to the maintenance of confidentiality that necessitate divulgence. Among these are:
1. Testifying in court
2. Reporting communicable disease
3. Reporting child abuse, spouse abuse, or elder abuse
4. Reporting gunshot or suspicious wounds if there is a reasonable cause to believe that the wound occurred as a result of a crime
5. Reporting for workers' compensation cases.

BREACH OF CONFIDENTIALITY
There may be situations in which there is an ethical demand for the physician to consider breaching patient confidentiality. Such a problem may occur when a patient who is HIV positive refuses to tell his or her spouse or significant other of the infection, thus placing the other at risk of contracting a lethal disease The physician who is aware of this is in a bind between duty to the patient and the stronger ethical demand to warn an unsuspecting person of significant danger. Such a breach is justified when all of the following conditions apply:

1. A high probability exists of serious physical harm to an identifiable person.
2. A likely benefit will result from breaking the confidence (for example, the harm can be prevented).
3. The breach is a last resort; persuasion and other approaches have failed.
4. The breach is generalizable; it would be reasonable for a doctor to breach your confidence and to treat you in the same way if you were the patient.

REFERENCES

Brennan TA. AIDS and the limits of confidentiality: the physician's duty to warn contacts of seropositive individuals. *J Gen Intern Med*. 1989;4:242-246.

Gostin LO et al. Privacy and security of personal information in a new health care system. *JAMA* 1993;270:2487-2493.

Health and Public Policy Committee of the American College of Physicians and Infectious Diseases Society of America. Acquired immunodeficiency syndrome. *Ann Intern Med*. 1986;104:575-581.

VI. HEART-LUNG DEATH

The centuries-old determination of death is the heart-lung standard. All 50 states recognize heart-lung death—the cessation of heartbeat and respirations—as death.

STEPS IN PRONOUNCING DEATH

When called to pronounce a patient dead, observe the following steps.

1. Ascertain code status.
2. Check for hypothermia or drug overdose, which can be confounding factors.
3. Auscultate for respirations and heart tones.
4. Check corneal reflexes with a wisp of cotton or tissue.

The patient is pronounced dead if no positive responses are found to any of the above. Document the time of death in the chart.

VII. BRAIN DEATH

By definition, "whole brain" death occurs when the entire brain—including the cerebral cortex and the brain stem—has died. This definition of death has been endorsed by the American Medical Association and the American Bar Association. It is law in 46 states.

CRITERIA FOR DIAGNOSIS
1. A neurologic event adequate to produce brain death
2. Reliable examination showing absence of brain-stem function.

FINDINGS ON PHYSICAL EXAMINATION
1. Profound coma—"eyes-closed unconsciousness"
2. No eye movement, no pupillary response
3. No corneal reflexes
4. No cough or gag reflex; no motor response to pain
5. No spontaneous respiratory attempts off the ventilator. (There are several ways of testing for apnea. If the patient is a potential organ donor, this test should only be done after consultation with the transplant coordinator.)

LABORATORY CONFIRMATION
1. Radionuclide tracer shows no cerebral blood flow.
2. Electroencephalogram (EEG) is not reliable, especially in cases of drug overdose or hypothermia.

LEGAL ASPECTS
If above criteria are satisfied, the patient is legally dead and no further treatment is necessary. It is important to document the time of death in the chart before turning off the ventilator.

HUMANITARIAN ASPECTS

Patients who are brain dead may not *look* dead. It is important to work with the family to help them acknowledge the death of their loved one. Occasionally, the ventilator needs to be left on for a slightly longer period to allow for this adjustment.

CONTROVERSIES

There is some current controversy about whether patients with cerebral cortical function loss but with a functioning brainstem (see section VIII on persistent vegetative state) should be included in an expanded definition of brain death. See also criteria of death in organ donation (section XIII).

REFERENCES

Halevy A, Brody B. Brain death: reconciling definitions, criteria, and tests. *Ann Intern Med.* 1993;119:519-525.

Veatch RM. The impending collapse of the whole-brain definition of death. *Hastings Cent Rep.* 1993;23:18-24.

VIII. PERSISTENT VEGETATIVE STATE (PVS)

DEFINITION
Total loss of cerebral cortical function with a functioning brain stem.

CHARACTERISTICS OF PVS
1. Sleep-like coma for a few days to a few weeks. Then the eyes open, and sleep-wake cycles begin.
2. "Eyes-open unconsciousness." Eyes move in random fashion but do not focus or follow. Patient is "awake but unaware." (In cases other than PVS, when recovery does occur, true tracking of objects by the eyes is often the first sign of recovery. This must be differentiated from a brief turning of the eyes of the PVS patient toward the source of sound, which is a primitive reflex.)
3. Unintelligible grunts, screams; grimacing and chewing without purpose. Swallowing is uncoordinated, so the patient must be tube fed.
4. Many reflexes are present including corneal, cough, gag, and startle.
5. The presence of gross involuntary, reflexive movement without purpose.

PROGNOSIS
After three months, the prognosis for recovery is virtually nil. It may be possible to establish lack of recovery of independent function after one month in patients whose PVS is caused by cerebral hypoxia.

DIAGNOSIS
The diagnosis is clinical; no definitive laboratory test is available. Neurological consultation should be obtained for confirmation. PVS is not recognized in law as "death."

MANAGEMENT

1. Good communication is required to help the family to understand that the patient, by definition, cannot be suffering. Sensations such as pain, hunger, thirst, and suffering—just like joy and awareness—are cortically mediated and are absent in PVS.

2. Usually the patient is not ventilator dependent, so the decision is whether to withdraw fluid and nutrition. This determination is easier to make if the patient has an advance directive or a reliable, informed surrogate decision maker.

FURTHER READING

Prognosis of PVS

One study reported that, following cerebral hypoxia-ischemia (the most common cause of PVS), no patient who remained vegetative for more than one month ever regained consciousness (*JAMA*. 1985;253:1420-1426). Some states require a period of three months in PVS for a definitive diagnosis.

The prognosis depends on the circumstances; in young adults and in cases of subarachnoid hemorrhage, it may take longer to predict the inability to recover independent function.

The general rules to establish a "hopeless" prognosis are:
*   3 months after hypoxic episode in child or young adult
*   12 months after head injury in a child
*   6 months after head injury in an adult.

After these intervals, recovery is extremely unlikely and those few who recover remain nursing-home patients with severe neurologic deficit, including the "locked-in" syndrome.

Prognosis in the Coma Phase Following Hypoxic-Ischemic Brain Injury

Patients who will not regain independent function have the following characteristics:
1. No pupillary light reflexes at time of initial exam
2. Lack corneal reflexes after the first day
3. Persistence of coma at seven days.

The absence of oculocephalic reflexes or the absence of purposeful motor response to pain portend a poor prognosis.

Laboratory Studies in PVS

Although there are no definitive studies, positron emission tomography (PET) scans of PVS patients have shown cortical glucose consumption to be at the same low level as that of patients in deep anesthesia. Serial computed tomography (CT) scans show significant and progressive atrophy but no specific changes. Autopsy studies routinely show bilateral hemispheric damage to a degree that is incompatible with consciousness.

REFERENCES

American Medical Association, Council on Scientific Affairs and Council on Ethical and Judicial Affairs. Persistent vegetative state and the decision to withdraw or withhold life support. *JAMA*. 1990;263:426-430.

Cranford RE. The persistent vegetative state: the medical reality (getting the facts straight). *Hastings Cent Rep*. 1988;18:27-32.

Levy DE, et al. Predicting outcome from hypoxic ischemic coma. *JAMA*. 1985;253:1420-1426.

IX. FUTILITY/UNREASONABLE PATIENT REQUESTS

NATURE OF REQUESTS

Sometimes patients make unreasonable requests: a computed tomography (CT) scan for a tension headache, penicillin for a viral infection, or laetrile for treatment of a malignancy. Ethical principles substantiate the physician's refusal to accede to a patient's demands to provide medical interventions that have no potential benefit or scientific merit—that is, those that are futile.

FUTILITY

Futility is difficult to define, but the following definition seems reasonable: "Medical futility means any effort to provide a benefit to a patient that is highly likely to fail and whose rare exceptions cannot systematically be reproduced" (Schneiderman and Jecker, 1995, p. 11).

Many ethicists believe that a distinction must be made between an *effect* that is limited to some part of the patient's body and the *benefit* that the patient has the capacity to appreciate and that improves the patient as a whole. For example, a ventilator that is effective in sustaining respiration may not be considered a benefit by a patient whose death from metastatic malignancy is imminent. Nonsentient patients (such as patients in a persistent vegetative state) cannot personally experience any intervention as a benefit.

The term *futility* refers to a specific medical intervention applied to a specific patient at a particular time. The term does not refer to a general situation of treatment or to a patient personally.

REASONS FOR REQUESTS FOR FUTILE OR IRRATIONAL THERAPY

1. *Unrealistic goals of the patient and/or family*: Physicians may fail to discuss achievable goals with the patient in terms of the change that would most likely result from the specific intervention being considered.
2. *Guilt*: Families may worry about betrayal of patient trust if they agree to withdrawal of treatment. They may also be compensating for past neglect or inattention.
3. *Confusion in formulation of the therapeutic plan*: This situation is most likely to occur in serious illness with a multiplicity of consultants (and no one apparently in charge).
4. *Mistrust of physicians by the patient or family*: Involvement of the primary care physician who knows the patient well may resolve this.
5. *Ethnic and socioeconomic differences*: Poor and minority patients may worry that any curtailment of services is rationing. They may be concerned about undertreatment as a form of discrimination.
6. *Denial mechanisms of the patient or family*: The patient or family may refuse to come to terms with reliable information.
7. *Misunderstandings/language barriers*: If an interpreter is necessary, he or she should be an objective observer, preferably with some medical training—not a family member.
8. *Religious issues*: Family is awaiting or certain of a miraculous cure.

RIGHTS OF PATIENTS

1. **Negative Rights (The Right of Refusal)**
   These are strong rights that include the right of the decisional patient to refuse any and all treatment. These rights are based on liberty and privacy. Physicians are obligated to respect such refusals.

2. **Positive Rights (The Right to Request a Specific Treatment)**

    These rights are weaker because they impose an obligation on others. Patients cannot demand treatment that is considered futile by the physician because this would obligate the physician to violate his/her professional integrity in order to provide the useless treatment.

GROUNDS FOR REFUSAL OF AN UNREASONABLE REQUEST

A doctor may refuse a patient's request for the following reasons:

1. The request is for something that is outside the scope of good medical care. Such a judgment is based on the lack of objective evidence for effectiveness of the requested intervention.
2. The request requires the doctor to act illegally.
3. The request requires the doctor to violate a personal and professional standard of responsible medical practice.
4. The requested treatment cannot be anticipated to produce any beneficial result for this patient.

ADDITIONAL CAVEATS

1. When the request is for treatment that has reasonable potential for both benefit and harm, the preference of the fully informed patient must take precedence.
2. Decisions should not be made solely on the basis of economic considerations.
3. Usually when the physician decides not to comply with a patient's request, a second opinion should be offered.

ETHICAL CONCERNS

1. "The right of the patient to choose does not imply the right to demand care beyond appropriate options based

on medical judgment and accepted standards of care, nor are physicians required to provide care in ways that in their personal judgment violate the principles of medical ethics" (*JAMA*. 1992;268:2282-2288).

2. "The well being principle circumscribes the range of alternatives offered to patients: informed consent does not mean that patients can insist upon anything they might want. Rather, it is a choice among medically accepted and available options, all of which are believed to have some possibility of promoting the patient's welfare" (President's Commission for the Study of Ethical Problems in Medicine and Biomedical and Behavioral Research. 1982:42-44).

LEGAL CONCERNS

The law does not outline the standards for clinicians to use to decide when to refuse an unreasonable patient request. Rather, the law articulates general duties that arise from the doctor-patient relationship and its ethical framework. The courts, through the laws of professional negligence, enforce these duties, maintaining that failure to fulfill them may result in compensable harm to the patient. The physician's primary legal duty is broad and nonspecific. He or she must possess and apply the knowledge and use the skill and care that is ordinarily used by reasonably well-qualified doctors in similar circumstances. This does not mean that the doctor must acquiesce to patients' demands that are unreasonable.

Many physicians unreasonably fear liability for not "doing everything," such as instituting every available technology if the patient requests it. The law rarely dictates the particulars of clinical practice and does not require that physicians do everything requested by a patient, agent, or guardian.

DIFFERENCE BETWEEN FUTILITY AND RATIONING

As Loewy points out, there is a danger that "futility" may be used as an excuse for decisions made on the basis of economic considerations—a real danger in a medical system driven by market forces.

It is particularly important to distinguish *futility*—a concept applied to a given patient and implying no apparent therapeutic benefit in that specific situation regardless of cost—from *rationing*—a concept that applies not to the individual but to society at large. Rationing also differs from futility in that it may acknowledge therapeutic benefit but deny it to some or all members of society because of cost factors.

THE CLINICIAN'S RESPONSE TO FUTILE SITUATIONS

It may be best to avoid the term *futility* in discussion with patients. One might instead use phrases such as "this won't help," or "this might even cause more problems." It is often better to approach discussions with patients in ways that will answer three questions:

1. What are the realistic goals of this particular patient in these particular circumstances?
2. Is the treatment being considered likely to achieve these goals without undue burden?
3. Is the planned intervention consistent with good medical practice?

Many requests for futile interventions result from incomplete or inadequate information. By spending time in careful communication with the patient (or surrogate) about reasonable expectations, the physician may avoid later confrontations. According to Paris: "If, after the physician has listened to the concern of family members (or the decisional patient) and explored the possibilities with them—including transfer of the patient to a willing physician—the family (or the decisional patient) persists in demands for continued life-prolonging treatment that the physician believes to be beyond well established medical criteria, the physician ought not to feel obliged to provide it. The physician's response in such cases should be: 'I'm sorry, but we don't do that here.' This is done not because the patient no longer has any value or because the physician lacks respect for the family's wishes. It is done because the obligation of physicians, as articulated in the Hippocratic oath, is to act for the benefit of the patient according to their ability and judgment." (*Cambridge Q.* 1993;2:147-149).

REFERENCES

American Medical Association, Council on Ethical and Judicial Affairs. Guidelines for CPR: ethical considerations in resuscitation. *JAMA*. 1992;268:2282-2288.

Loewy EH, Carlson RA. Futility and its wider implications. *Arch Intern Med.* 1993;153:429-431.

Paris JJ. Pipes, colanders, and leaky buckets: reflections on the futility debate. *Cambridge Q.* 1993;2:147-149.

President's Commission for the Study of Ethical Problems in Medicine and Biomedical and Behavioral Research. *Making Health Care Decisions: The Ethical and Legal Implications of Informed Consent in the Patient-Physician Relationship.* Washington, DC: US Government Printing Office; 1982:42-44.

Schneiderman LJ, Jecker NS. Is the treatment beneficial, experimental or futile? *Cambridge Q.* 1996;5:248-256.

Schneiderman LJ, Jecker NS. *Wrong Medicine.* Baltimore, Md: Johns Hopkins University Press; 1995.

Wear S, Logue G. The problem of medically futile treatment: falling back on a preventive ethics approach. *J Clin Ethics.* 1995;6:138-148.

X. THE DIFFICULT PATIENT

Some patients are very difficult to care for in a professional manner. They may engender feelings of anger, rejection, frustration, or resentment on the part of the physician. Taking care of such patients requires specific skills.

SPECIFIC SITUATIONS

1. The Seductive Patient

Physician response: At first naiveté, then confusion and embarrassment.

Management tips:

1. Always have another person present, especially for pelvic or genital exams.
2. Be wary of accepting gifts.
3. Be suspicious of frequent phone calls, especially after hours.
4. Terminate relationship if necessary.

2. The Chronic Somatizer

Physician response: Initially impatience, later rejection.

Management tips:

1. Establish a long-term, "one-doctor" relationship.
2. Schedule frequent (every six to eight weeks), short visits.
3. Examine thoroughly if new symptoms arise.
4. Avoid unnecessary diagnostic procedures.
5. Minimize medication use.
6. Refer to psychiatrist or psychologist when appropriate but maintain ongoing relationship as primary therapeutic manager.

3. The Manipulating Drug Abuser

Physician response: Anger.

Management tips:

1. Set limits and stick to them.
2. Never prescribe narcotics for someone else's patient.
3. Be suspicious of strange stories about lost pills.
4. Refer to pain clinic or detox program if patient is willing.

4. The Overly Dependent Patient

Physician response: Gratification at first, then resentment.

Management tips:

1. Be wary of the patient with extreme gratitude.
2. Set firm limits for frequency of visits and calls.
3. Freely acknowledge to the patient your own human limitations.

5. The Terminally Ill Patient

Physician response: Impotence and frustration.

Management tips:

1. Realize that these patients are looking for care, not cure.
2. Avoid specific prognostic parameters.
3. Ensure that adequate comfort care measures are maintained.
4. Make an effort to be there for the patient.

6. The Noncompliant Patient

Physician response: Loss of control, then loss of interest.

Management tips:

1. Recognize limitations in changing patient's behavior.
2. Resist the desire to give up.

3. Change therapeutic plan to modalities that the patient will accept, realizing that you may have to settle for less than optimal treatment.

7. The Borderline Personality

Physician response: Anger and hostility.

Management tips:

1. Refer for psychiatric co-care, but be aware of "splitting."
2. Avoid drugs that are addictive.
3. Set firm limits and be consistent.

SKILLS AND TECHNIQUES NEEDED TO MANAGE DIFFICULT PATIENTS

Physicians who are adept at managing difficult patients point out that when physicians avoid acknowledging these feelings, they are more likely to misdiagnose or mismanage the patient. Recommendations include:

1. Stop disavowing intense or hateful feelings toward a patient.
2. Recognize that these feelings are, in a sense, part of the "diagnosis" for that particular patient.
3. Discuss feelings with colleagues in order to obtain their help.
4. Remember that, ultimately, it is not these feelings but how the physician behaves toward the patient that is most important.
5. Most patients need a stable, long-term relationship with a primary care physician who is not compelled to evaluate all symptoms extensively.

REFERENCES

Barsky AJ. Hidden reasons some patients visit doctors. *Ann Intern Med*. 1981;94:492-498.

Drossman DA. The problem patient. *Ann Intern Med*. 1978;88:366-372.

Groves JE. Taking care of the hateful patient. *N Engl J Med*. 1978;298:883-887.

XI. PAIN CONTROL/PALLIATIVE CARE

THE NEED FOR MORE AGGRESSIVE TREATMENT
Many patients and family members fear that pain control may be inadequate (with good reason). The prevalence of this fear may be responsible, in part, for the increasing interest in euthanasia and assisted suicide.

MISTAKES THAT ARE MADE
1. The drug selection may be poor. For example, meperidine (Demerol®) is clearly inferior to morphine for the control of the severe pain of bony metastases.
2. The dose may be inadequate or the dosing interval too long. For example, 75 milligrams of Demerol® every four hours for postoperative pain in a 210-pound man is insufficient.
3. Physicians may fear causing addiction in patients who experience chronic pain or terminal illness and have to take large doses for long periods of time.
4. Physicians may prescribe inadequate doses of narcotics to patients who are terminally ill, for fear of inducing respiratory depression.

GOOD PAIN MANAGEMENT
1. Choice Dose of Drugs
Learn the appropriate drugs for given clinical situations and the proper dose and dosing interval.
2. Knowledge about Addiction
Addiction (true psychological dependence) is rare in patients who receive narcotics for pain, even if the drug must be continued for protracted periods. Tolerance—the need to increase the dose for the same pharmacologic effect—varies from patient to patient. Physiologic dependence occurs in all patients with long-term use, but opio-

ids can be tapered over several days to avoid withdrawal symptoms.

3. Respiratory Depression

Hospices and oncology services report that respiratory depression is uncommon in patients who are receiving opioids for the control of pain; if present, it is often from some cause other than the opioid. Pain itself is a respiratory stimulant, and the opioid effect on the respiratory center diminishes rapidly with chronic use. If the patient is terminally ill and the dose of opioid required to produce comfort does happen to depress respiration, it is still reasonable to allow the undesired effect (respiratory depression) in order to achieve the desired effect (relief of suffering).

4. Terminal Sedation

Physicians may have to resort to this procedure to relieve the suffering of a dying patient whose disease is incurable and whose symptoms are refractory (cannot be controlled despite aggressive efforts that do not compromise consciousness). Symptoms requiring deep sedation for relief include:

- Dyspnea (most common cause)
- Pain not controlled by opioid without distressing side effect
- Agitated delirium, restlessness with myoclonus
- Unrelieved vomiting.

FURTHER READING

Hennepin County, Minnesota, Medical Society Policy Statement

"The administration of large quantities of narcotic analgesics is not euthanasia when the purpose is to alleviate pain and suffering, not to shorten the life of the patient. There are sufficient ethical, moral and medical reasons to prescribe morphine and other pain relieving medications even at the risk of hastening the patient's death.

The goal of treatment is to relieve patient suffering to the fullest extent possible. For dying patients there is no 'cap' dose; high doses may be required for the relief of pain and suffering."

From Wanzer et al

"In the patient whose dying process is irreversible, the balance between minimizing pain and suffering and potentially hastening death should be struck clearly in favor of pain relief. Narcotics and other pain medications should be given in whatever dose and by whatever route is necessary for relief. It is morally correct to increase the dose of narcotics to whatever dose is needed, even though the medication may contribute to the depression of respiration or blood pressure, the dulling of consciousness or even death, providing the primary goal of the physician is to relieve suffering. The proper dose of pain medication is the dose that is sufficient to relieve pain and suffering, even to the point of unconsciousness."

REFERENCES

Buchan ML, Tolle SW. Pain relief for dying persons: dealing with physicians' fears and concerns. *J Clin Ethics*. 1995;6:53-61.

Cherny NL, Portenoy RK. Sedation in the management of refractory symptoms: guidelines for evaluation and treatment. *J Palliative Care*. 1994;10:31-38.

Melzack R. The tragedy of needless pain. *Scientific American*. 1990;262:27-33.

Quill TE, Lo B, Brock DW. Palliative options of last resort. *JAMA*. 1997;278:2099-2104.

Rousseau P. Terminal sedation in the care of dying patients. *Arch Intern Med*. 1996;156:1785-1786.

Wanzer SH, et al. The physician's responsibility toward hopelessly ill patients: a second look. *N Engl J Med*. 1989;320:844-849.

XII. AUTOPSY

NEED FOR AUTOPSIES

Physicians sometimes think autopsies are no longer necessary in this era of computed tomography and magnetic resonance imaging. Autopsies are still needed, however, for medical, legal, epidemiological, and familial reasons.

INDICATIONS FOR AUTOPSY

1. Comply with medical examiner's requirements.
2. Clarify puzzling cases.
3. Delineate suspected or unsuspected medical conditions.
4. Provide useful information to the family.
5. Reassure survivors with negative findings.
6. Collect statistical data.
7. Define environmental and occupational hazards.
8. Provide legal and forensic information.
9. Enhance clinical, pathological, and medical education.

MEDICAL EXAMINER CASES

These are cases that must, by law, be reported to the medical examiner:

1. Unexplained or unusual circumstances surrounding death
2. All homicides
3. All suicides
4. All deaths following abortion
5. All deaths due to poisoning (homicidal, suicidal, or accidental)
6. All deaths following accidents, regardless of whether the injury was the primary cause of death (For example, a patient hospitalized for treatment of fractures sustained in an automobile accident who dies in the hospital of a myocardial infarction still needs to be reported.)

7. When no physician is in attendance
8. When the attending physician refuses to sign the death certificate
9. If there is doubt about the need to report, it is best to call the medical examiner's office.

NOTIFYING AND COUNSELING THE FAMILY
Immediately after pronouncing death:

1. Notify the attending physician and determine if he or she wishes to inform the family.
2. If the task is delegated to you, speak in person to the family, if possible. Phone only if necessary.
3. Identify yourself as the doctor caring for their loved one.
4. Inform them gently and avoid euphemisms such as "passed away" and "expired."
5. Express sympathy. Physical contact such as a hand on the shoulder may be appropriate.
6. If appropriate to the situation, you may wish to involve the hospital chaplain and/or the social worker.
7. Quietly and sensitively raise the question of autopsy, giving the reasons for its importance in this case (such as uncertainty of diagnosis, the family's need to know, scientific advancement).
8. Assure family that there is no cost to them and that an open-casket funeral service is not precluded by the procedure.

OBTAINING CONSENT FOR AN AUTOPSY
Consent for the autopsy must be obtained in writing, by telegram, or by fax. The hospital will pay the costs for the telegram. Phone consent is not valid. Consent should be obtained from the next of kin in the following order:

1. Surviving spouse. If none, then
2. Adult children. If none, then

3. Parents. If none, then
4. Brothers and sisters. If none, then
5. Any relative (or friend) who assumes custody of the body.
6. If none of the above can be found 48 hours after death, hospital administration can give consent.

If the case is reported to the medical examiner and accepted for autopsy, family consent is not necessary; the family has no option for refusal. Furthermore, a consent signed by any agent listed above does not preclude an autopsy by the medical examiner.

AFTER THE DEATH (NO AUTOPSY DONE)

1. You may want to attend the funeral (if your relationship to the patient makes this appropriate).
2. Always send a card or a brief letter or make a follow-up call.
3. If possible, have the surviving caregiver return to the hospital for a follow-up conversation; this is a good time to resolve any questions or concerns.

AFTER THE DEATH (AUTOPSY DONE)

1. Same as above.
2. Your follow-up call should include information about the preliminary autopsy report. The pathologists are also available for consultation.
3. Written autopsy reports are usually available within four to six weeks of the procedure. A copy can be given to the family personally or by letter.

REFERENCES

Gonzalez C. The influence of culture in the authorization of an autopsy. *J Clin Ethics*. 1993;4:192-194.

Orlowski JP, Vinicky JK. Conflicting cultural attitudes about autopsies. *J Clin Ethics*. 1993;4:195-197.

Perkins HS, Supik JD, Hazuda HP. Autopsy decisions: the possibility of conflicting cultural attitudes. *J Clin Ethics*. 1993;4:145-154.

XIII. ORGAN DONATION

SUITABLE DONORS
1. Under age 75 for solid organs
2. Under age 70 for bone and soft tissue donation
3. No age limit for eye donation.

TRANSPLANTABLE ORGANS
Kidney, liver, heart, lung, pancreas, and small bowel.

TRANSPLANTABLE TISSUES
Skin, long bone, heart valve, vein, and eye.

CRITERIA FOR ORGAN DONATION
1. Solid organ donors must meet the criteria for brain death (section VII, page 23) and must be on ventilator support.
2. The issue of non-heart-beating cadaver donors (NHBCD) remains controversial but is current policy at some institutions. In these patients, Regitine® is given in the operating room to increase organ perfusions and the ventilator is discontinued. Hypotension, apnea, and cardiac standstill ensure, and the patient is pronounced dead by heartlung death criteria. Organ procurement ensues immediately. This protocol blurs some of the clear lines established by brain-death protocols—thus the controversy.
3. Bone and tissue donation occurs within 24 hours of asystole.
4. Eye donation occurs within four to six hours of asystole.
5. Patients with infection, sepsis, or malignancy are not candidates for organ donation.
6. These criteria are quite flexible; more organs and tissues from older donors are used now than in the past.

CONSENT FOR ORGAN DONATION

1. A signed donor card takes precedence over the wishes of any survivor. These wishes should be explained to the family.
2. The family of any potential donor (who does not have a specific contraindication to donation) must be asked about donation and should be encouraged to give permission (especially when the patient is brain dead and is thus a suitable donor for solid organs).
3. Even if the person did not sign the driver's license for organ donation, the family may agree to donate organs.
4. Technically, the body of a dead person becomes the property of the next of kin, so organ donation cannot be specified in an advance directive. For order of priority of next of kin, see section XII, pages 41 and 42.

COST OF ORGAN DONATION

Families need to be told that they are not responsible for any of the costs related to organ donation for transplant.

FUNERAL ARRANGEMENTS AFTER ORGAN DONATION

Assure the family that the body is released soon after the organs or tissues are removed and that funeral arrangements are rarely delayed. When donation is complete, prosthetic replacements are used to restore the body to its natural appearance. Open-casket viewing is possible with any type of donation.

INSTITUTIONAL RESOURCES

All institutions with transplant programs have someone with expertise in organ procurement who can give advice. A phone call to the coordinator on call is recommended before approaching the next of kin for permission.

REFERENCES

American Medical Association, Council on Ethical and Judicial Affairs. Ethical considerations in the allocation of organs and other scarce medical resources among patients. *Arch Intern Med*. 1995;155:29-40.

Cohen C, Benjamin M. Alcoholics and liver transplantation. *JAMA*. 1991;265:1299-1301.

Moss AH, Siegler M. Should alcoholics compete equally for liver transplantation? *JAMA*. 1991;265:1295-1298.

Ubel PA, Arnold RA, Caplan AL. Rationing failure: the ethical lessons of retransplantation of scarce vital organs. *JAMA*. 1993;270:2469-2474.

Youngner SJ, Arnold RM. Ethical, psychological, and public policy implications of procuring organs from non-heart beating cadaver donors. *JAMA*. 1993;269:2769-2774.

XIV. AIDS

Ethical dilemmas encountered in the care of patients with acquired immunodeficiency syndrome (AIDS) include issues of compassion, medical futility, care of the incompetent patient, confidentiality, and management of the difficult patient (see also sections IV, V, IX, and X).

PHYSICIANS' RESPONSE TO THE AIDS RISK

Health professionals' fear of contracting AIDS will exist as long as there is a risk that the human immunodeficiency virus (HIV) can be transmitted in the healthcare setting. Despite infection control procedures, a very small (much less than 1 percent) occupational risk exists. This risk requires a professional response: physicians have always had to set aside personal fears in order to take care of sick persons.

The physician may also have to overcome personal antipathies to patients of different cultural and socioeconomic background (such as intravenous drug users) and different sexual orientations. If a gap exists between doctor and patient, ethical discussions regarding medical indications, the patient's preferences, allocation of resources, use of cardiopulmonary resuscitation (CPR), and treatment in the intensive care unit (ICU) are made more difficult.

The American Medical Association Council on Ethical and Judicial Affairs has stated, "A physician may not ethically refuse to treat a patient whose condition is within the physician's current realm of competence solely because the patient is sero-positive. Persons who are sero-positive should not be subjected to discrimination based on fear or prejudice" (*JAMA*, 1988;259:1360-1361). Federal laws contain similar conditions.

RECOMMENDATIONS

1. Most patients with HIV infection benefit from combined drug therapy, which requires highly specialized clinical knowledge. For this reason, most HIV-positive patients are followed by infectious disease specialists. Because primary care physicians are often involved in the initial diagnosis and management, they should learn as much about the disease as possible.

2. In many cases, doctors must try to bridge the social or psychological gap between themselves and their patients.

3. New treatment regimens have decreased the morbidity and mortality of HIV infection, and AIDS is now becoming more of a chronic rather than a terminal disease.

4. Sometimes, however, treatment becomes futile; the physician should then withdraw or withhold the treatment, using the skills and paradigms described in this text. Encouraging the patient to complete an advance directive helps decision making in these circumstances (see sections I, II, and XVII).

REFERENCES

American Medical Association, Council on Ethical and Judicial Affairs. Ethical issues involved in the growing AIDS crisis. *JAMA*. 1988;259:1360-1361.

Derse AR. HIV and AIDS: legal and ethical issues in the emergency department. *Emerg Med Clin North Am*. 1995;13:213-223.

Haas JS, et al. Discussions of preferences for life-sustaining care by persons with AIDS. *Arch Intern Med*. 1993;153:1241-1248.

Steinbrook R, et al. Ethical dilemmas in caring for patient with the acquired immunodeficiency syndrome. *Ann Inter Med*. 1985;103:787-790.

Wachter RM, Luce JM, Hopewell PC. Critical care of patients with AIDS. *JAMA*. 1992;267:541-547.

Zuger A, Miles SH. Physicians, AIDS, and occupational risk: historic traditions and ethical obligations. *JAMA*. 1987;258:1924-1928.

XV. PEDIATRIC ISSUES

STANDARDS: BEST INTEREST VERSUS SUBSTITUTED JUDGMENT

One of the most difficult aspects of making decisions regarding the treatment of children is knowing what is in the best interest of the child. Nonetheless, this is the appropriate standard for decision making. Parents should be involved in this process. The substituted-judgment standard cannot generally be employed in cases involving children because, unlike adults, pediatric patients have never possessed decision-making capacity. The wishes of older children should be considered in decision making, and some children who are "mature minors" (see section IV, page 17) can be treated like adults.

THE PEDIATRICIAN AS CHILD ADVOCATE

The primary role of the attending pediatrician is that of child advocate. Reasonable medical measures that are in the best interest of the child should be employed, with at least a trial of treatment even in the most critically ill children. As in adult medicine, futility may be a contraindication to continued treatment in some cases.

Pediatricians have encouraged immunization, Head Start, nutrition programs, and other innovative initiatives to improve the lives of children. Pediatricians have clearly demonstrated that adequate food and housing, proper sanitation, and childhood immunizations are more potent overall lifesavers than technical medical interventions.

ADVISING PARENTS

As advisors to the parents of their patients, pediatricians can counsel and support them as they reach decisions regarding the best interest of their child.

This is a difficult process, for the physician must be as objective as possible in giving an opinion or medical recommendation. The pediatrician may fail in the role of advisor in two ways. He or she may hide behind the "objectivity" of the medical facts and refuse to give any guidance on what is medically and ethically correct, merely saying "These are the options. What do you want me to do?" Conversely, the physician may knowingly or unknowingly manipulate the parents into making the decision the physician prefers by relating only those facts that would support that particular decision.

It is useful to give the parents time and to encourage them to get a second or even a third opinion in difficult circumstances. If the ethical issues remain unclear, a consultation with the ethics committee may be appropriate.

NEONATAL INTENSIVE CARE

In the past, medical care for critically ill newborns was mainly supportive. Data collected in the neonatal intensive care unit (NICU) confirm that gains have been made in the survival of infants with increasingly low birth weights. The limit for providing ventilatory support in the 1960s was 1500 grams; in the 1990s the limit is 500 grams.

The success, however, is not unqualified. Ventilatory management has been difficult, and multiple complications may occur. The low-birth-weight neonate may have patent ductus arteriosus, immature brain and germinal matrix, and incomplete retinal vascularization. Increased attention and funding of neonatal intensive care technology may be diverting attention and funding from basic prenatal care. As is true in adult medicine, the recent focus on high technology is threatening the traditional primary care focus of pediatrics.

ETHICAL ISSUES

Neonatal ethical issues focus on the aggressiveness of treatment and resuscitation of infants who are already being treated aggressively in the NICU. Pediatric ethics issues for the mature minor mirror those of the adult patient. The capacity of children to be involved in decisions depends upon their age and intellectual capacity.

REFERENCES

Harrison H. Principles for family centered neonatal care. *Pediatrics*. 1993;92:643-650.

Jonsen AR, Siegler M, Winslade WJ. *Clinical Ethics*, 3rd ed. New York: McGraw-Hill; 1992.

Lantos JD, et al. Providing and forgoing resuscitative therapy for babies of very low birth weight. *J Clin Ethics*. 1992;3:283-287.

President's Commission for the Study of Ethical Problems in Medicine and Biomedical and Behavioral Research. *Deciding to Forego Life-Sustaining Treatment*. Washington, DC: US Government Printing Office; 1983.

XVI. ETHICS AND MANAGED CARE

Most physicians are involved with managed care organizations (MCOs) full time or at least part time. Managed care and capitation have introduced new stresses into the practice of medicine and into the relationship between doctor and patient.

NEW PRESSURES ON PHYSICIANS

1. Divided Loyalties

The traditional role of the physician as patient advocate has to be balanced against the need to save money for the organization. The major question is whether the physician can function in this role without compromising patient care and patient welfare.

2. Limited Tests and Treatments

The American Medical Association Council on Ethical and Judicial Affairs has issued the following statement: "As part of the process of giving patients informed consent to treatment, physicians should disclose all available treatment alternatives, regardless of cost, including those potentially beneficial treatments that are not offered under the terms of the plan" (*JAMA*. 1995;273:330-335).

Patients need to be aware that limitations of interventions (testing and treatment) should be dictated by their disease process rather than by the rules of the MCO. If a second-best but less expensive antibiotic is prescribed because of the restrictions of the MCO formulary, patients need to know this (and accept it).

3. Limited Choice of Physician/Specialist Referral

One real benefit of managed care systems may be the establishment of a primary care physician who provides continuity of care, serves as a ready source of contact, and makes appropriate referrals for care beyond his or her expertise.

Problems can occur if the primary care physician does not have ongoing responsibility (for example, if the patient sees a different physician at each visit); if the primary care physician is pushed beyond his or her level of expertise in order to avoid expensive referral, or if the primary physician is allowed to refer only to MCO physicians when a far superior specialist for a particular problem is in the community but not associated with the MCO.

PROBLEMS INHERENT IN THE MANAGED CARE ORGANIZATION

1.   Administrative Costs and Profit Taking

Most MCOs are for-profit entities with stockholders who must be paid. In such MCOs, about 74 percent of revenues are returned to healthcare; the remainder goes to investor profits, administrative costs, and executive salaries. More than $50 billion was generated as profits in healthcare in 1997. This money is unavailable for medical needs at a time when policy makers solemnly agree that we "can't afford" universal healthcare.

2.   Patient and Doctor "Churning"

Patients are moved from doctor to doctor and system to system. Sometimes a patient may be forced to change healthcare systems several times even while employed at the same job. Similarly, doctors and healthcare organizations join and leave MCOs abruptly. All of these changes disrupt the patient-doctor-clinic-hospital relationship.

3.   Confidentiality

Preservation of confidentiality of patient information is increasingly difficult with computerized records moving in and between organizations.

4.   Provision of Care of the Indigent or Support for Medical Education or Research

MCOs, with a few notable exceptions, lack an educational mission and avoid involvement with teaching hospitals and institutions that provide care for indigent patients.

PRACTICE GUIDELINES

Guidelines must be flexible, scientifically legitimate, and widely accepted by professional medical organizations. Guidelines should remain *guidelines* and not become *requirements*. They should allow for some variability to accommodate unique clinical circumstances, because patients often do not present with classical textbook symptoms and do not fit neatly into protocols.

Practice guidelines can be very helpful in avoiding marginally useful or unhelpful interventions and tests. However, they can also become restrictive, and have been referred to as "cookbook medicine." Guidelines must be reassessed and revised periodically by physicians to avoid becoming outdated recipes.

RATIONING

Macro-allocation deals with the way resources are allocated to groups of people—to the entire MCO or to society as a whole. The lives involved are faceless and statistical. *Microallocation* refers to the situation in which people deal with one another on a one-to-one basis; the lives are identified lives. Rationing at this level is "bedside rationing." According to the American Medical Association, allocation judgments about costs and services that approach a "rationing" decision (such as the denial of a procedure that benefits a patient) are not part of the physician's traditional role and, indeed, conflict with it (*JAMA*. 1995;273:330-335).

Physicians should not be involved in the process of micro-allocation. At the bedside or in the clinic on a one-on-one basis, the only responsibility of the ethical physician is to act as an advocate for the patient. If distribution is to be fair and just, rationing decisions must be made by society so that any limits the physician imposes on his/her patients are shared by all physicians and patients in the same clinical setting.

On the other hand, physicians should be involved in the process of macro-allocation. It is their duty as good citizens—

a duty made even more important by the special knowledge physicians bring to the deliberations. Physicians abrogate their public responsibility if they allow bureaucrats or nonprofessional individuals to make policy decisions without their emphatic input.

CAN THE ETHICAL PHYSICIAN-PATIENT RELATIONSHIP ENDURE IN THE MANAGED CARE MILIEU?

The answer can be yes, but only under certain conditions.

1. The MCO should allow full informed consent: the patient should be informed of all appropriate interventions for his or her problem including those not offered by the MCO contract.

2. Physicians' salaries should not be individually predicated only on saving the MCO money, but also on the quality of care rendered. If there is a small incentive bonus, it should be truly small and patients should be aware of it.

3. If there are MCO practice guidelines, there should be allowance for deviation under unusual circumstances and frequent physician-directed revision to reflect new scientific evidence.

4. The MCO should have a medical board composed of participating physicians who are responsible for periodically reviewing restrictions on services to subscribers and other issues related to healthcare coverage as well as quality of care.

5. In short, the participating physicians must be allowed as much latitude as possible in exercising their primary responsibility—fulfilling the trust of their patients that physicians' acts are motivated only by concern for patients' welfare.

FURTHER READING

The Patient-Physician Covenant

The following statement was written by a group of medical ethicists and endorsed by the American College of Physicians and the American Board of Internal Medicine:

Medicine is, at its center, a moral enterprise grounded in a covenant of trust. This covenant obliges physicians to be competent and to use their competence in the patient's best interests. Physicians, therefore, are both intellectually and morally obliged to act as advocates for the sick wherever their welfare is threatened and for their health at all times. Today, this covenant of trust is significantly threatened. From within, there is growing legitimation of the physician's materialistic self interest; from without, for-profit forces press the physician into the role of commercial agent to enhance the profitability of health care organizations. Such distortions of the physician's responsibility degrade the physician-patient relationship that is the central element and structure of clinical care.

To capitulate to these alterations of the trust relationship is to significantly alter the physician's role as healer, carer, helper, and advocate for the sick and for the health of all.

By its traditions and its very nature, medicine is a special kind of human activity—one that cannot be pursued effectively without the virtues of humility, honesty, intellectual integrity, compassion, and effacement of excessive self interest. These traits mark physicians as members of a moral community dedicated to something other than its own self interest.

Our first obligation must be to serve the good of those persons who seek our help and trust us to provide it. Physicians, as physicians, are not, and must never be, commercial entrepreneurs, gate closers, or agents of fiscal policy that runs counter to our trust. Any defection from primacy of the patient's well being places the patient at risk by treatment that may compromise quality of or access to medical care.

We believe the medical profession must reaffirm the primacy of its obligation to the patient through national, state, and local professional societies; our academic, research, and hospital organizations; and especially through personal behavior. As advocates for the promotion of health and support for the sick, we are called upon to discuss, defend, and promulgate medical care by every ethical means available. Only by caring and advocating for the patient can the integrity of the profession be affirmed. Thus we honor our covenant of trust with patients.

Reprinted with permission from Crawshaw R, et al. The patient-physician covenant. *JAMA*. 1995;273:1553. Copyright 1995, American Medical Association.

REFERENCES

American Medical Association, Council on Ethical and Judicial Affairs. Ethical Issues in managed care. *JAMA*. 1995;273:330-335.

Crawshaw R, et al. The patient-physician covenant. *JAMA*. 1995;273:1553.

Daniels N. *Just Health Care*. New York: Cambridge University Press; 1985.

Ginsberg E, Ostow M. Managed care: a look back and a look ahead. *N Engl J Med*. 1997;336:1018-1020.

Gostin LO, et al. Privacy and security of personal information in a new health care system. *JAMA*. 1993;270:2487-2493.

Jecker NS, Jonsen AR. Healthcare as a commons. *Cambridge Q*. 1995;4:207-216.

Kassirer JP. Is managed care here to stay? *N Engl J Med*. 1997;336:1013-1014.

Kerr EA, et al. Primary care physicians' satisfaction with quality of care in California capitated medical groups. *JAMA*. 1997;278:308-312.

Swartz K, Brennan TA. Integrated health care, capitated payment and quality: the role of regulation. *Ann Intern Med*. 1996;124:442-448.

Weingarten S. Practice guidelines and predication rules should be subject to careful clinical testing. *JAMA*. 1997;277:1977-1978.

XVII. ADVANCE DIRECTIVES

DEFINITION

An advance directive (AD) is a statement a patient makes, while still in possession of decision-making capacity, about how treatment decisions should be made at some future time if he or she loses the capacity to make such decisions.

TYPES OF AD

1. Living will (LW) statutory form
2. Power of attorney for health care (PAHC) statutory form
3. Nonstatutory forms.

LIVING WILL

1. Provisions

Most statutory forms are documents stating the desire to die a "natural" death and not to be kept alive by medical treatment and machines. In many states, the principal may also stipulate that fluid and nutrition are to be discontinued in the event of persistent vegetative state (PVS).

2. Activation

Usually the LW becomes effective on the determination of "terminal" illness or "imminent" death (death expected within six months) or the diagnosis of PVS made by two physicians.

POWER OF ATTORNEY FOR HEALTHCARE

1. Provisions

Most statutory forms provide a way for the principal to appoint a person to act as healthcare agent, proxy, or surrogate to make healthcare decisions in the event that the principal loses the capacity to make decisions. The PAHC allows the principal to add specific directions, and often the agent may be given authority to have feeding tubes withheld or withdrawn (even in the absence of PVS).

2. Activation

The PAHC becomes effective when two physicians, or one physician and one psychologist, determine that the principal is no longer decisional.

PREFERENCE

Patients may ask for the physician's advice about ADs. The statutory form of the PAHC is the best choice because it allows all of the options of a LW and has the added advantage of providing an agent—someone who knows the principal well and can take an active role in the decision-making process on the patient's behalf. The PAHC also allows for the addition of specific instructions to the agent. There is no advantage to filling out both forms. *Note: The laws regarding LWs and PAHCs vary from state to state. It is wise to check the provisions and standards for activation in your own jurisdiction.*

FURTHER READING

Living Will
Strengths
1. Allows the physician to understand the patient's wishes and motivations.
2. Extends the patient's autonomy, self-control, and self-determination.
3. Relieves the patient's anxiety about unwanted treatment.
4. Relieves physician's anxiety about legal liability.
5. Reduces family strife and sense of guilt.
6. Improves communication and trust between patient and physician.

Weaknesses
1. Applicable only to those in PVS or the terminally ill (patients who have a disease that is incurable and will die regardless of treatment).
2. Death must be imminent (likely to occur within six months).
3. Ambiguous terms may be difficult to later interpret.
4. There is no proxy decision maker, so:
   - It requires prediction of final illness scenario and available treatment.
   - It requires physician to make decisions on the basis of an interpretation of a document.

Note: In light of these weaknesses, it is strongly recommended that patients complete the PAHC and not the LW. There is no advantage to having both.

Power of Attorney for Healthcare (PAHC)
Activation of PAHC

Lack of decision-making capacity must be certified by two physicians or one physician and a psychologist who have examined the patient. Until then, the patient makes all the decisions.

Advantages

1. Physician has someone to talk with—a proxy, a knowledgeable surrogate—who can provide a substituted judgment of how the patient would have chosen. If the agent is unable to provide a substituted judgment, the agent and physician together can use the best-interest standard (how a reasonable person might choose in consideration of the benefit-burden concept of proportionality).
2. Provides flexibility; this decreases ambiguity and uncertainty because there is no way to predict all possible scenarios.
3. Authority of agent can be limited as person desires.
4. Avoids family conflict about rightful agent.
5. Provides legal immunity for physicians who follow dictates.
6. Allows appointment of a nonrelative (especially valuable for persons who may be alienated from their families).
7. Most forms can be completed without an attorney.
8. Principal may add specific instructions to the agent such as the following: I value a full life more than a long life. If my suffering is intense and irreversible, or if I have lost the ability to interact with others and have no reasonable hope of regaining this ability even though I have no terminal illness, I do not want to have my life prolonged. I would then ask not to be subjected to surgery or to resuscitation procedures, or to intensive care services or to other life-prolonging measures, including the administration of antibiotics or blood products or artificial nutrition and hydration (adapted from Bok).

Nonstatutory Forms

These are forms that are not codified in state law. They may contain ambiguous language, which can cause difficulty in interpretation. In many states, nonstatutory forms—unlike the statutory forms of the LW and PAHC—may not provide legal immunity for physicians who follow the dictates of the document.

Patient Self-Determination Act (PSDA)

This federal law, which went into effect in 1991, involves all Medicare and Medicaid providers (hospitals, nursing homes, hospices, and health maintenance organizations).

According to the provisions of the Patient Self-Determination Act (PSDA), all healthcare providers must:

1. Give all patients written information at the time of admission, advising them of their rights to refuse any treatments and to have an AD. This is usually done by nursing or social service staff shortly after admission, but patients may ask physicians about ADs.
2. Document the presence of an AD in the patient's record.
3. Have written policies respecting the rights of patients to have an AD and to refuse treatment.
4. Make provisions to educate staff and community regarding these issues.
5. Prohibit discrimination against a person because they do or do not have an AD.

Some Misconceptions Patients Have about ADs

1. *"If I sign one, I can't change my mind."* An AD can easily be revoked—orally, in writing, or by filling out a new AD that supersedes the old.
2. *"I'm young and/or I'm in good health, so I don't need an AD."* The *Cruzan* and *Quinlan* cases—two prominent court cases that drew attention of the public to this issue—involved women in their twenties.
3. *"If I have an AD, paramedics would not resuscitate me."* Because the standard of activation for the LW is the presence of a terminal condition and for the PAHC is loss of decision-making capacity, these documents, as a rule, do not speak to emergency situations; insufficient time exists to determine the presence of the effective activating elements. An occasional exception is the chronically ill individual who specifies do not resuscitate in the PAHC.
4. *"My family might not want me to sign an AD."* Families generally welcome the opportunity to discuss these issues, and the presence of an AD can do much to relieve family guilt if it becomes necessary to withdraw or withhold treatment.
5. *"My spouse/family knows what I want"* or *"My physician knows what I want."* Numerous surveys report that neither family members nor physicians are accurate in their estimation of patients' preferences; designation of an agent with specific instructions is the best way to circumvent this problem.

Some Misconceptions Physicians Have about ADs

1. *"The provisions of the AD may require me to act counter to my philosophy and conscience."* The physician needs to discuss the AD with the patient to make sure that no conflict exists between the patient's desires and the physician's principles. If a conflict is present, it may be necessary to transfer the patient to the care of another physician.

2. *"I know what my patients want."* See item 5 above.
3. *"I can't bill for the time spent discussing these ADs."* This is an important obligation, regardless of the financial reward. However, the service can usually be billed under the codes for counseling, patient education, and preventive care.

Recommendations to Patients and the Public Regarding ADs

1. Think about the issues and your specific wishes; discuss them with family.
2. Complete the PAHC form rather than the LW form.
3. Discuss your desires fully with both the primary and alternate agents. You may want to add some written instructions.
4. Discuss the decisions with your personal physician to get agreement on specifics.
5. These documents need to be circulated widely. Copies of the document should be given to primary and alternate agents, close family members, personal physician, and personal attorney.

Recommendations to Physicians

1. It is the physician's responsibility to initiate discussion with all decisional patients, regardless of age. This is best done in the office (clinic) at a nonthreatening time. Use of printed informational material is helpful, as is the availability of PAHC forms in the office.
2. Describe the settings in which an AD is important. Tell patients that you, as their physician, will be in a better position to direct their treatment with a written AD.
3. Assure patients that symptomatic care and treatment will never be withheld.
4. Patients may need time to reflect and discuss these issues with their families. It may be a good idea to initiate the topic at one clinic visit and to discuss it further at a later visit.
5. Document a patient's oral statements if an AD is not completed. If an AD is completed, file it in the patient's record.
6. Review the AD with the patient to prevent misunderstandings.
7. Emphasize the need for the patient to discuss the AD fully with his or her family.
8. Complete an AD (PAHC) yourself.

REFERENCES

Bok S. Personal directions for care at the end of life. *N Engl J Med.* 1976;295:362-369.
Caralis PV, et al. The influence of ethnicity and race on attitudes toward advance directives, life-prolonging treatments, and euthanasia. *J Clin Ethics.* 1993;4:155-165.

Emmanuel LL, et al. Advance directives for medical care: a case for greater use. *N Engl J Med*. 1991;324:889-895.

Gillich MR, et al. Medical technology at the end of life: what would physicians and nurses want for themselves? *Arch Intern Med*. 1993;153:2542-2547.

Lo B. Improving care near the end of life: why is it so hard? *JAMA*. 1995;274:1634-1636.

Lynn J, et al. Perceptions by family members of the dying experience of older and seriously ill patients. *Ann Intern Med*. 1997;126:97-106.

Miles SH, Koepp R, Weber EP. Advance end-of-life treatment planning. *Arch Intern Med*. 1996;156:1062-1068.

Pearlman RA, et al. Insights pertaining to patient assessments of states worse than death. *J Clin Ethics*. 1993;4:33-41.

Pearlman RA, Uhlmann RF, Jecker NS. Spousal understanding of patient quality of life: implications for surrogate decisions. *J Clin Ethics*. 1992;3:114-120.

XVIII. ETHICS CONSULTATION

ETHICS COMMITTEES

Institutional ethics committees (ECs) have many different configurations. Many are standing committees of the medical staff, which report to the medical executive committee or governing staff of the hospital. Most meet monthly, or more frequently as occasion demands. Typically ECs have three tasks:

1. Education—of committee members, staff, and community
2. Policy formulation—the EC is not a policy-making body but will suggest policy on request of the medical staff or hospital administration
3. Case consultation—on request.

REASONS FOR CASE CONSULTATION

An ethics consultation might be considered for some of the following reasons:

1. For clarification of issues regarding decision-making capacity, informed consent, or advance directives
2. To provide recommendations for cases involving do-not-resuscitate orders or withdrawal of treatment
3. To help in resolution of ethical conflict—between family and caregivers, patient and caregivers, patient and family, or among staff members.

FURTHER READING

Case Consultation Method

(This is the approach used by the authors' institutional EC.)

1. **Response to Consultation Request**

   The consultant or the EC member who initially responds to the request for consultation should consider the following:

   a. Who requested the consult? If it was not the attending physician, does he or she agree?

b.   What is the ethical problem? Is the problem ethical—or does it involve legal, social, or psychological issues; staff conflict; or miscommunication? Is it a problem that needs referral to another service?

c.   What specifically is being requested of the EC? Clarification of the problem? Mediation? Recommendations?

2.   Evaluation by the Responding Consultant

a.   See the patient. If patient has decision-making capacity, notify him or her of the nature of the visit.

b.   Interview nursing personnel, other personnel, and family members.

c.   Discuss the problem with the attending physician and other consultants.

d.   Review the chart.

3.   Decision about Emergency Meeting of Full EC

a.   If the problem is uncomplicated, common, and the reaction of the EC can be anticipated, the consultant may resolve it.

b.   If the problem is unusual, problematic, delicate, or has legal ramifications, a full emergency EC meeting is called.

Assessment of the Ethical Problem

(By either the initial consultant or the entire EC)

1.   Medical Facts

a.   Decision-making capacity of the patient

b.   Current medical status, diagnosis, and prognosis

c.   Recommended treatment and reasonable alternative treatments

d.   Effect of no treatment

e.   Assessment of the patient's life expectancy

f.   Views of caregivers.

2.   Patient's Preference

a.   Has the patient been informed and given time to reflect on options?

b.   What are the patient's personal/social factors? What is his or her value system?

c.   What is the patient's personal assessment of quality of life?

d.   What are the patient's current expressed choices?

e.   Are there any advance directives?

3. External Factors

a. Family
- How well do they know and represent the patient?
- Do they understand the situation? Are they in agreement?
- Is there any conflict of interest?
- If there is no advance directive, who is the decision maker?

b. Religion—are religious or cultural values involved?

c. Expense—is it a factor in the patient's decisions?

d. Legal issues
- Are there applicable hospital policies or state statutes?
- Is there potential liability?

Problem Resolution

1. Make sure the information is complete.
2. Delineate the ethical problem clearly.
3. Clarify the options.
   a. Did we assure as much patient autonomy as possible?
   b. Are our recommendations consistent with the patient's preferences or best interest?
   c. Are our recommendations consistent with ethical principles?

Reporting

1. Recommendations are made as recommendations. It is up to the attending physician to take or reject them, as is true of all consultations.
2. Report of the consultation will be placed on the chart, if requested.
3. Full report of the consultation will be detailed in the minutes of the EC for educational purposes, but special care will be taken to preserve patient confidentiality.
4. Full minutes as required by medical staff bylaws will go to the medical staff executive committee.

Follow Up

In many situations, the consultant will need to follow the patient in order to be available for further consultation. In this way, the consultant can check on the patient's status and make progress reports to the EC for educational purposes.

REFERENCES

Fletcher JC, Siegler M. What are the goals of ethics consultation? a consensus statement. *J Clin Ethics*. 1996;7:122-126.

Jonsen AR. Case analysis in clinical ethics. *J Clin Ethics*. 1990;1:63-65.

La Puma J, Schiedermayer D. *Ethics Consultation: A Practical Guide.* Boston: Jones and Bartlett; 1994.

Singer PA, Pellegrino ED, Siegler M. Ethics committees and consultants. *J Clin Ethics.* 1989;1:263-267.

Walker MU. Keeping moral spaces open: new images of ethics consulting. *Hastings Cent Rep.* 1993;23:33-40.

XIX. EUTHANASIA AND ASSISTED SUICIDE

DEFINITIONS

1. **Euthanasia**

    The physician participates in an intentional, deliberate act to cause the immediate death of a person with terminal, incurable, or painful disease by the medical administration of a lethal drug.

2. **Assisted Suicide**

    The physician provides the lethal drug with instructions for its use but is not the agent. The patient decides when and if to use the drug.

    Most, but not all, ethicists agree that euthanasia and assisted suicide differ from one another significantly because of the agency. In euthanasia the physician is the direct agent; in assisted suicide it is the patient who is the direct agent.

LEGAL ASPECTS

Euthanasia is illegal in all states. Suicide is not illegal, but all states except Oregon now have some sort of legal prohibition against assisted suicide. In 31 states there is a specific law against assisting a suicide; in the remaining 18 states, prosecution is possible under other existing statutes.

ETHICAL ASPECTS

1. American Medical Association policy: "The intentional termination of the life of one human being by another is contrary to public policy, medical tradition, and the most fundamental measures of human value and worth" (AMA, *Euthanasia*).

2. American College of Physicians Ethics Manual: "Although a patient may refuse a medical intervention and the physi-

cian may comply with this refusal, the physician must never intentionally and directly cause death or assist a patient to commit suicide" (*Ann Intern Med.* 1989;111:245-335).

STATE INITIATIVES

Initiatives placed before the people of Washington in 1991 and California in 1992 to allow physician-assisted death failed in both states by relatively close margins. A ballot measure in Oregon to allow physician assistance in suicide for suffering patients with terminal illness passed in 1994. It was never implemented because of legal challenge. Oregon voters in 1997 reaffirmed support (60 to 40) and the federal appeals court lifted the injunction. Thus, Oregon is the only state in which physician-assisted suicide (but not euthanasia) is legal.

Lower federal court decisions in California and New York that declared the state statutes against assisted suicide unconstitutional were appealed to the U.S. Supreme Court. The Court considered both decisions together and rendered a unanimous decision that the state statutes against assisted suicide did not violate either the "due process" or equal protection provisions of the 14th Amendment of the U.S. Constitution. Thus, the two federal court decisions were negated. The opinions of several Supreme Court justices affirm the following:

1. The right of competent patients to discontinue or to withhold any treatment, even that considered life sustaining
2. The right of competent patients to receive sufficient medication to relieve pain, even if that dose causes shortening of the patient's life
3. The right of competent patients whose suffering cannot otherwise be relieved to have terminal sedation
4. Because none of the above actions are considered suicide, physicians who accede to such patient requests cannot be considered to be "assisting a suicide."

The Court also allowed that the issue is not settled and that individual state legislatures might in the future take action legitimizing assisted suicide. Further attempts will undoubtedly follow. Because this issue will not go away, physicians as a group need to consider thoughtfully the professional response to this situation.

THE PHYSICIAN'S RESPONSE

It is the responsibility of caring physicians to analyze the stimuli for these initiatives that have such widespread public support and to attempt to change those factors that are amenable to change. Prominent public fears that fuel this debate are:

1. The concern that the pain experienced by a terminally ill patient will not be controlled adequately
2. The worry about loss of control and the indignity of dependence during the final illness
3. The concern that medical technology will continue to be used inappropriately, thus delaying an "easy" death.

By providing adequate pain control to terminally ill patients without fearing addiction or respiratory depression, physicians will help assuage the first concern. Use of appropriate palliative measures and increased reliance on hospice care will relieve many of the other concerns. By strongly recommending the use of advance directives and discussing these issues with their patients, physicians can reduce the burden of end-of-life decision making.

If all of these interventions are carried out successfully, the stimulus for state initiatives should decrease. However, regardless of the effectiveness of good pain control and palliative care, there will remain a small but significant group of patients for whom no alternative to death is acceptable and for whom aid in dying is not irrational. Each physician will have to decide for himself or herself what the appropriate response will be.

REFERENCES

American College of Physicians. Ethics manual, part I: history, patient, other physicians. *Ann Intern Med*. 1989;111:245-335.

American Medical Association, Council on Ethical and Judicial Affairs. Decisions near the end of life. *JAMA*. 1992;267:2229-2233.

American Medical Association, Council on Ethical and Judicial Affairs, *Euthanasia*. Chicago: American Medical Association; June 1988. Report 12:1-40.

Brody H. Assisted death: a compassionate response to a medical failure. *N Engl J Med*. 1992;327:1384-1388.

Brody H. Causing, intending, and assisting death. *J Clin Ethics*. 1993;4:112-117.

Miller FC. A communitarian approach to physician assisted death. *Cambridge Q*. 1997;6:78-87.

Orentlicher D. The legalization of physician assisted suicide. *JAMA*. 1996;335:663-667.

Quill TE, Cassel CK, Meier DE. Care of the hopelessly ill: proposed clinical criteria for physician assisted suicide. *N Engl J Med*. 1992;327:1380-1383.

Quill TE, Lo B, Brock DW. Palliative options of last resort: a comparison of voluntarily stopping eating and drinking, terminal sedation, physician-assisted suicide, and voluntary active euthanasia. *JAMA*. 1997;278:2099-2104.

XX. THE PHYSICIAN'S PROFESSIONAL RESPONSIBILITIES

THE FUNDAMENTAL GOALS OF MEDICINE

The general goals of medicine include the following:

1. Prevention of disease and untimely death
2. Cure of disease, when possible
3. Improvement or maintenance of functional status when cure is not possible
4. Palliation (relief of pain and suffering), pursuit of a peaceful death, and comfort care in all situations
5. Patient education and counseling.

Good clinical judgment requires a realistic understanding of the goals of treatment in a particular case. Physician and patient together should determine which goals are actually possible. Often a doctor and patient can agree that the goal should be palliation and comfort. Unfortunately, both physician and patient often fail to acknowledge the need to change goals when cure becomes impossible.

THE DOCTOR'S DUTIES

The central responsibility of the clinician is to use his or her technical expertise to respond to a patient's request for help by:

1. Making an accurate diagnosis of the patient's condition
2. Informing and educating the patient about the diagnosis
3. Recommending the course of action the clinician considers to be best
4. Discussing the benefits and risks of this course and of reasonable treatment alternatives
5. Discussing prognosis if treated or untreated
6. Carrying out with technical skill the necessary diagnostic and therapeutic procedures
7. Assuring the patient that he/she will not be abandoned.

INDIVIDUALIZING TREATMENT

In making a recommendation about clinical care, physicians need to evaluate the individual patient in terms of:
1. The patient's comprehension and self-understanding
2. The organic seriousness of the condition
3. The seriousness of the condition in the patient's eyes
4. The need for urgent action
5. The physical, psychological, and social impact of the options on the patient
6. The ability of the patient to participate in his or her own care
7. The patient's values, beliefs, fears, and hopes.

MORAL DECISION MAKING

Clinicians are responsible for reaching a decision that is not only clinically and technically sound but is also morally appropriate and suitable for the specific problems of the particular patient being treated. The medical (technical) aspects of the decision answer the question, "What *can* be done for this patient?" The moral component involves patient wishes and answers the question, "What *ought* to be done for this patient?"

REWARDS

Quill and Cassel summarize the rewards of medicine: "Clinical medicine is ultimately a humbling and exhilarating profession, filled with joy, sorrow, and an overabundance of uncertainty that comes with establishing a genuine long-term connection with patients. To practice medicine with a commitment to caring and to be there no matter what the future holds is to experience the richness of the human condition over and over again and to know one has made a difference" (*Ann Intern Med.* 1995; 122:373).

REFERENCES

McCullough LB. John Gregory (1724-1773) and the invention of professional relationships in medicine. *J Clin Ethics*. 1997;8:11-21.

Peabody FW. The care of the patient. *JAMA*. 1927;88:877-882.

Pellegrino ED. Toward a reconstruction of medical morality: the primacy of the act of profession and the fact of illness. *J Med and Philosophy*. 1979;4:32-56.

Quill TE, Cassel CK. Non-abandonment: a central obligation for physicians. *Ann Intern Med*. 1995;122:368-374.

Specifying the goals of medicine. *Hastings Cent Rep*. November-December 1996; 26 (special supplement):9-16.

Tumulty PA. What is a clinician and what does he do? *N Engl J Med*. 1970;283:20-24.